How to Build a Monstrous Physique

For the Extreme Hardcore Bodybuilder

Nekoterran

From the Author:

I want to thank you and congratulate you for purchasing the book How to Build a Monstrous Physique: For the Extreme Hardcore Bodybuilder.

This program contains proven steps and strategies on how to build a monstrous physique.

In this program, you will learn unmatched wisdom in bodybuilding that doesn't exist anywhere else.

Note: This program is part of a trio. The information in this program doesn't function in isolation. To successfully build a monstrous physique, the participant must first master *How to Build More Muscle than Ever Before* and *Intestinal Cleanse and Reconstruction* before attempting the monstrous program. I hope you not only read the information, but take action on the knowledge to obtain maximum results in bodybuilding.

Note #2:

It is possible that your current clothes will not fit after a few weeks into the monstrous program.

Also be aware that achieving a monstrous physique may stir envy from other bodybuilders, including physical trainers at your local gym. If small-minded individuals attack you→ do not fight back or attempt to straighten out their thinking. Just know you are well on your way to building a monstrous physique!

Thanks again for purchasing this book. I hope you not only read but apply the information as well.

CONTENTS:

If you enjoy this book do consider leaving a review...

www.nekoterran.com/advice

Read together with…

Basic Internal Detox

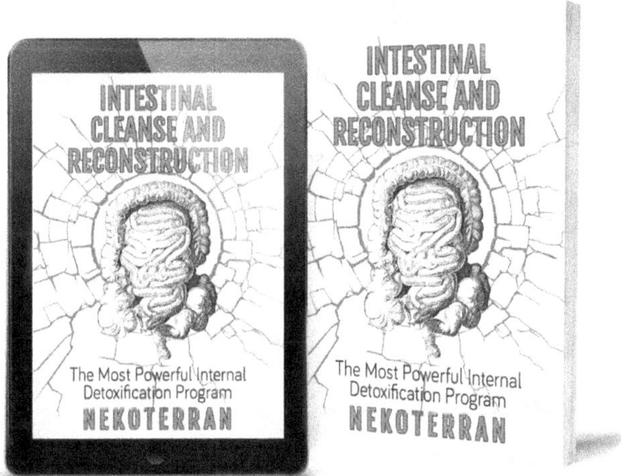

✓ Deep internal detoxification program.

✓ This is the ideal program to begin with.

✓ Complete this program first before attempting weight loss or bodybuilding basics

✓ Works in conjunction with every other program.

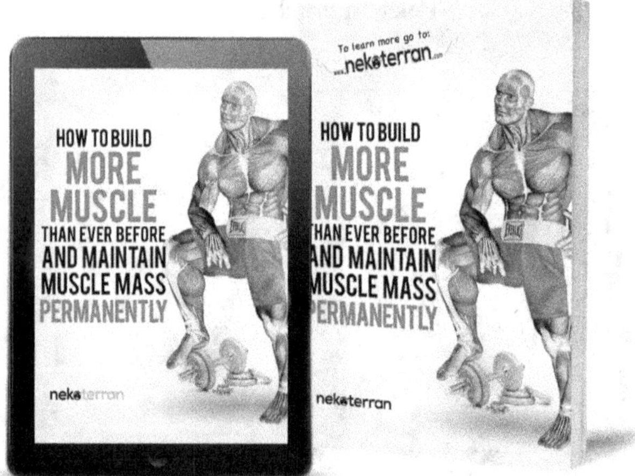

- ✓ What builds muscles.
- ✓ What causes muscle mass deterioration.
- ✓ What causes body fat.
- ✓ How to burn body fat.
- ✓ How to maintain muscle mass.
- ✓ How to maintain a fat-less physique.
- ✓ Choose only basic bodybuilding or basic weight loss.

Introduction:

I am not a fitness instructor, nor do I have a coaching license.

The information in this program is not tailored to replace your current workout routine or diet. This program has not been evaluated by the AFAA, Medical Fitness Association, American Sports and Fitness Association, IDEA Health & Fitness Association or any other fitness association.

All the information you will learn is based on direct experience and experimentation on myself, my bodybuilding peers, fitness enthusiasts and the average out-of-shape individual who also achieved outstanding results.

However, it is possible that the techniques outlined have some measure of risk, like everything in this world. You have to use common sense and consult with your physician or fitness instructor if necessary prior to the workouts and dietary principles. You, the reader alone, is the only one responsible for the methods outlined in this e-book.

Before we move on...

Let me make one thing absolutely clear from the start:

I am not interested in advertising supplements,

nor am I pushing anyone to buy supplements.

Some or most of the nutrients listed here have to be taken externally. Meaning our bodies cannot produce them on its own. From foods alone, nutrients are impossible to be absorbed.

My only interest is for you to achieve your health/fitness goals after having come across my program.

This program is means serious business, and only those who are dedicated can follow.

Back to business…

COMPLETE THE DETOX AND MUSCLE PROGRAMS FIRST

Why cleanse and reconstruct the intestines first?

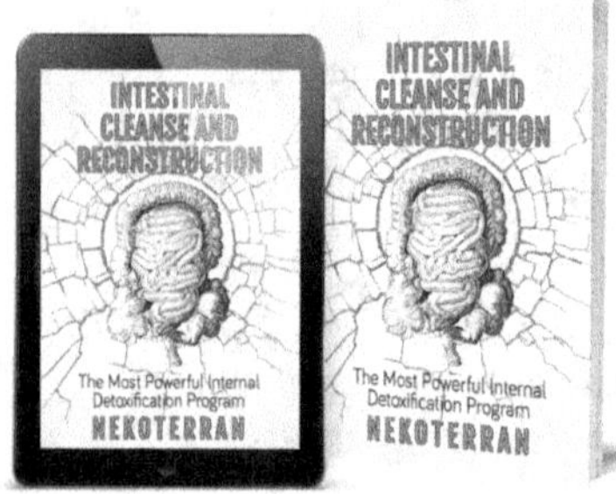

The bowels are one of the primary channels of elimination. What do the intestines and bowel movements have to do with health, fitness, weight loss and bodybuilding? The bowels have everything to with health, fitness, weight loss and bodybuilding!

Like the analogy of a dishwashing machine from my weight loss and bodybuilding programs…once a set of dishes is fully washed, the old set must be removed for a new set of dishes to begin a new washing cycle. If you don't have a bowel movement first thing in the morning, and 30 - 40 minutes after every meal, you are chronically constipated!

Cleaning out the bowels of undesired pollution will keep the system clean and improve digestion.

And what builds muscles?

Digestion builds muscles!

Probiotics can be even more successfully transplanted once the mucoid plaque, unfriendly bacteria and all unnecessary gunk have been cleaned out of the intestines.

Note: Cleansing and reconstruction of the intestines + transplanting friendly bacteria BEFORE commencing any bodybuilding program is the ideal place to start. Building muscle mass or a monstrous physique comes second. Digestion and absorption will be easier and faster, and so will building muscles.

Why master how to build more muscles before the monstrous program?

In my first bodybuilding programs, I explain what to eat, what builds muscles, how to maintain muscle mass, what causes body fat, and everything you need to build a large muscular physique. The How to Build a 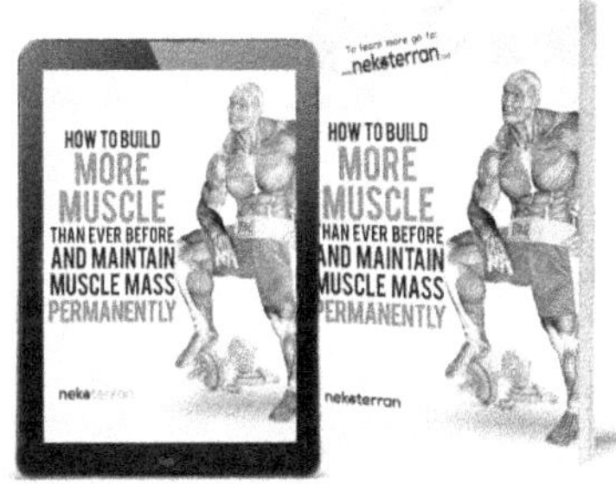 Monstrous Physique program is an addition or part 2 of the bodybuilding book. This program only focuses on building a monstrous physique and does not explain the basics of bodybuilding.

Why is building a monstrous physique the final step of the trio?

Like I said, the monstrous program functions synergistically as a team with the other two programs. The monstrous program isn't the most difficult; intestinal cleansing is. However, the workout section here is a little bit more complex/hardcore than the first bodybuilding program.

WHAT IT TAKES TO BUILD A MONSTROUS PHYSIQUE

Now you don't have any excuses.

A powerful top-of-the-line blender is absolutely necessary to build a monstrous physique.

The best investment you can possibly make is to purchase a high-quality blender.

What are green drinks?

Green drink is another name for vegetable juice and grass juice.

Any non-starchy vegetable is great to juice with a pinch of lime or stevia to improve the taste.

How many lemons have to be squeezed for one drinking glass? 5-6 lemons or more?

The point is, by juicing vegetables, large quantities of vegetables that cannot possibly be consumed in solid form can be consumed in juice form. Never underestimate the power of juicing. A highly alkaline internal environment will boost energy and maintain a clean internal system.

Alkaline body pH levels, the internal environment established inside the intestines, is crucial for health, internal detoxification, weight loss, bodybuilding…everything! If you keep your vehicle (body) clean; the disease, body fat, loss of muscle, aging (oxidation), mucoid plaque buildup will be reduced and parasites, molds, and fungal overgrowth will not be able to survive. Alkaline pH levels cannot be emphasized enough. And of course, a deep internal detoxification will go a long way in keeping the system clean.

Purchasing a quality blender can be a life-changing event. Juicing green drinks or juicing anything else and pretty much cooking overall will never be the same experience from this point onwards.

Most cheap/average blenders break down, burn out, and overheat the vegetable juices. As you will learn, if the vegetable juices are heated, enzymes within the raw plants will die.

Choose a blender of your choice.

FREE shipping.

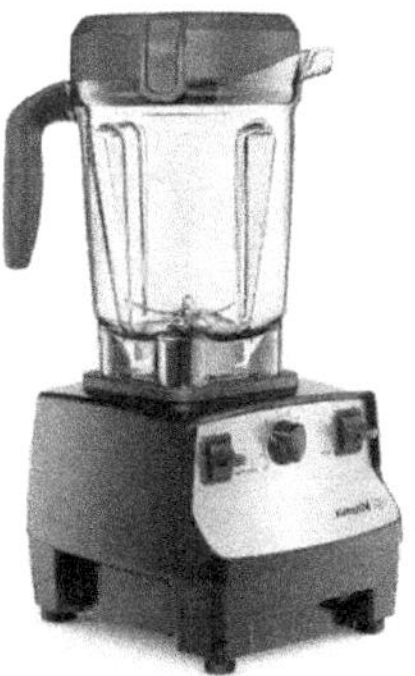

Certified Reconditioned- 5300 $299

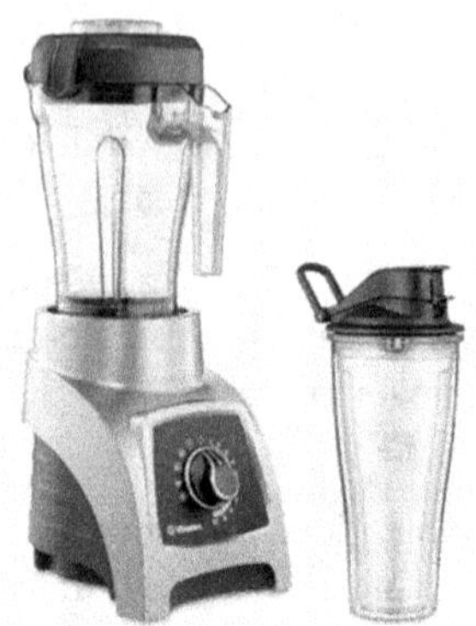

Personal- S30 $329

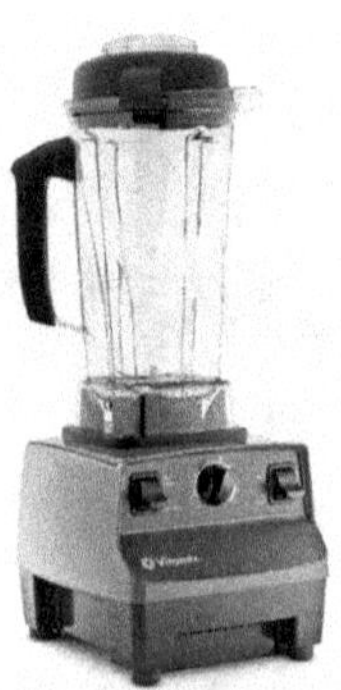

Legacy (food blender) - 5200 $449

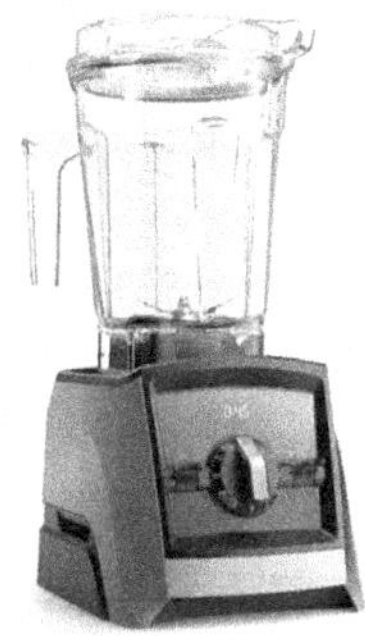

Ascent Series A2300 $469

Some chain names that use Vitamix:

Starbucks, Beans Bins, Jamba Juice, Jugo Juice, Booster Juice, Lavazza Coffee, Tully's, Costa Coffee, Robeks, Maui Wowi Hawaiian Coffee & Smoothies, Smoothie King, Mr. Smoothie, Orange Julius, Tropical Smoothie Café, and the list goes on.

The feature I like the most about the Vitamix blender is that the motor is extremely powerful and will never overheat the vegetable juices, keeping the **enzymes** alive. The only downside I can think of is that the motor is loud and heavy.

Note: It's true that I recommend green drink powders as a replacement for green juices. However, blending vegetables directly using a high quality blender cannot even be put in the same category **quality**-wise by using a super blender.

What builds muscles?

Digestion builds muscles.

Digestion happens in the stomach.

If digestion is strong + fast + easy = building muscles will be strong + fast + easy.

As you have learned, eating a fresh piece of ginger after or before a meal will fire up digestion x2. Here, I will teach you how to fire up digestion many times over.

Enzymes

What is an enzyme?

Enzymes are stimulants to chemical reactions. Enzymes speed up the chemical reactions within the body. Enzymes cause digestion. Fat, protein, and carbohydrate metabolism are chemical reactions. Enzymes have to come from food or must be directly produced by the body.

Cooked foods of any kind have zero enzymes. Raw vegetables, fruits and green drinks are totally packed with enzymes. You will notice that your body will digest and pass out raw vegetables quickly. The reason is because of enzymes.

If you are consuming 2/3 of overall intake of food raw and only 1/3 cooked combined with green drinks or blended green drinks, then you have plenty of enzymes required for digestion. Again, what is eaten doesn't builds muscles; digestion is what builds muscles. How the food is eaten is more important than what foods are eaten.

Enzymes are fragile. Exposure to heat, sunlight or oxygen can damage, if not strip off, a large portion of enzymes from the plant. An average blender will overheat the vegetable juices, destroying all the enzymes. **The whole point of drinking green drinks is to provide enzymes and maintain alkaline pH levels in the system!**

In addition, combining the completion of the deep internal detoxification program with enzyme supplements in between meals with water will fire up digestion many times over. And if you are in a restaurant where the majority of the foods will be cooked, take some enzyme supplements to speed up digestion.

Here are 2 of my favorite enzyme supplements that have delivered the best results to build muscle mass.

Choose only one supplement from each category.

All natural supplements are listed in:

www.nekoterran.com/supplements

(take 3 caps, 2-3 times a day in green drinks + amino acids)

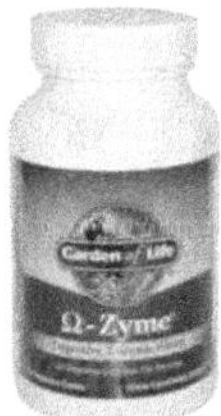

Garden of Life, Omega-Zyme, Digestive Enzyme Blend, 90 Caplets Omega-Zyme
$28.99

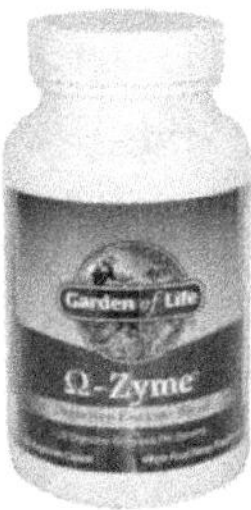

Garden of Life, Omega-Zyme, Digestive Enzyme Blend, 180 Veggie Caplets $44.09

Basic building blocks

Amino acids are the building blocks of life.

L-glutamine is the most abundant amino acid found in the human body.

The human body requires amino acids to

- Enhance digestion
- Repair body tissue
- Repair damaged bowel lining (leaky gut)
- Reduce inflammation in intestinal lining
- Protect intestinal walls and repels irritants
- Repair and regenerate muscles after strenuous usage

Synthesize and protect muscle tissue

- Produce glycogen and immune support
- Be a source of energy and stamina

Amino acids have multiple benefits for digestion, bowels, muscle repair, muscle building, and fat loss. Think of amino acids as the absolutely necessary supplement that feeds on muscles and burns body fat.

The body produces amino acids. L-glutamine mostly comes from plants such as cabbage, beets, parsley, beans and spinach. You can never overdose on amino acids; negative effects from amino acids are almost unheard of.

By combining L-glutamine (plant based) together with amino acids from white fish, you will be able to build a monstrous physique that you did not know was even possible to accomplish.

(Take 3 caps, 3 times a day in green drinks **together** with 1 tea spoon of l-glutamine 3 times a day.)

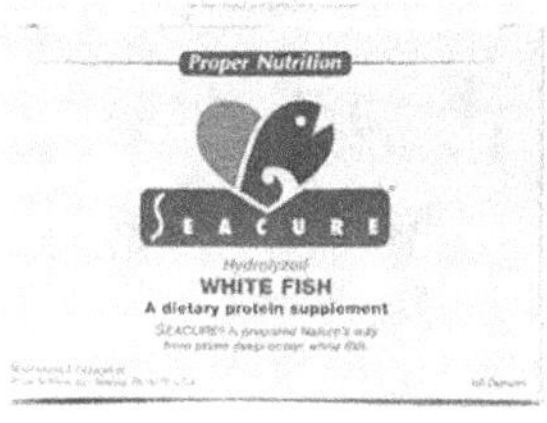

Proper Nutrition SeaCure in Blister Packs - 180 Capsules **$36.98**

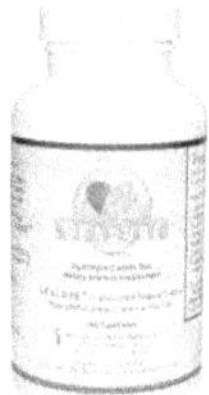

Proper Nutrition SeaCure in Blister Packs - 180 Capsules **$35.73**

http://www.propernutrition.com/

The importance of friendly bacteria

Note: Friendly bacteria is crucial for extreme hardcore bodybuilders.

Friendly bacteria are also fragile. By cleaning out and reconstructing the intestines, transplanting friendly bacteria, keeping an alkaline green environment within, and consuming inulin in stevia, you should keep the friendly bacteria alive for long periods of time. **Without friendly bacteria fully colonized in the bowel walls, all the nutrients and supplements consumed will go to waste.** The best way to keep the existing friendly bacteria expanding, and continuously add more probiotics is by kefir in goat milk.

2nd option: After transplanting friendly bacteria by caplets, I like to consume probiotics in powder form with my green drinks daily. Not as intense as before, only 1-2 teaspoons a day.

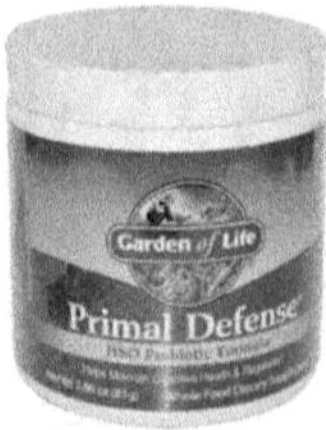

Garden of Life, Primal Defense, Powder, HSO Probiotic Formula, 2.86 (81 g) **$33.99**

Note: Kefir granules mixed in goat's milk is more powerful than taking primal defense. Your first choice should be to find kefir and goat's milk. The same text from the detox program is posted here.

Goat milk and Tibetan kefir mushrooms

What KIND of milk harms or doesn't harm the bones?

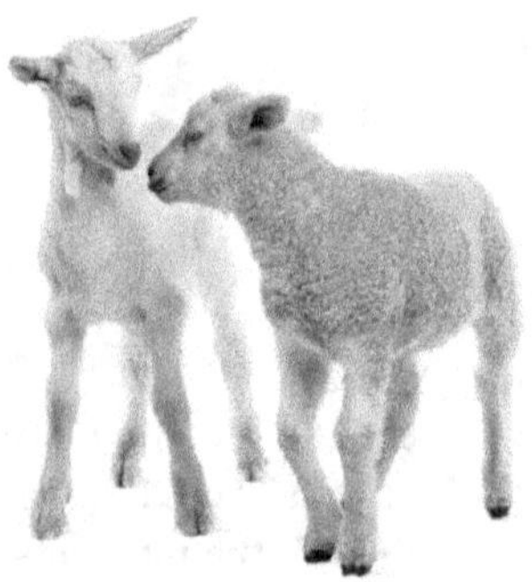

Milk in its natural form is raw milk, and it is put in the category of alkaline drinks. The milk 99% of people drink, bought from the supermarket that has been pasteurized and homogenized, is acidic.

Unpasteurized, non-homogenized milk is the milk that provides all the nutrients to the bones and body. Pasteurized milk found in the grocery stores and supermarkets has been heated to kill bacteria. This is the milk that harms the bones, causes allergens, etc.

Cow milk is extremely difficult for the stomach to digest. And in many cases, it causes inflammation. Cows have four stomachs, and they function nothing like a human's. Cow milk and all processed dairy products from the grocery store simply are inconsumable.

Know that there is a healthier alternative for cow milk. Goat milk is packed with nutrients, such as copper, zinc, magnesium, calcium, and vitamins A, B2, C, D, and it tastes pretty much the same as cow milk.

Goat milk carries A2 protein, which is the closest to human breast milk. Goat milk is easy to digest, lower in lactose, doesn't carry the allergens cow milk contains, and is low in casein protein. Protein congests the system and is hard to digest. The casein protein in cow milk causes allergies, inflammation, bowel irritations, leaky gut syndrome, and a whole lot of gastrointestinal issues. High levels of medium-chain fatty acids found in goat milk converts to energy instead of storing as excess body fat.

Where can raw, unpasteurized, non-homogenized goat milk be purchased?

Finding raw goat milk can be extremely challenging. But once you find a quality supplier, the supply of goat milk will be well worth the effort.

Raw goat milk won't be available in any kind of supermarket or grocery store. Depending in which country you live in, the best way to find raw goat milk is to do an internet search. If you cannot find it on the internet, you will most likely have to contact a dairy company/factory directly, and if not, go to a farm with goats and ask for some raw milk.

Where can Tibetan kefir mushrooms be purchased?

Kefir mushrooms are
fairly easy to find and cost-
effective.

Depending where your
located, you will have to
find the grains on the
internet. Kefir grains are
living organisms. All you have to do is purchase the grains
once, re-supply the goat milk and the grains will multiply over
time.

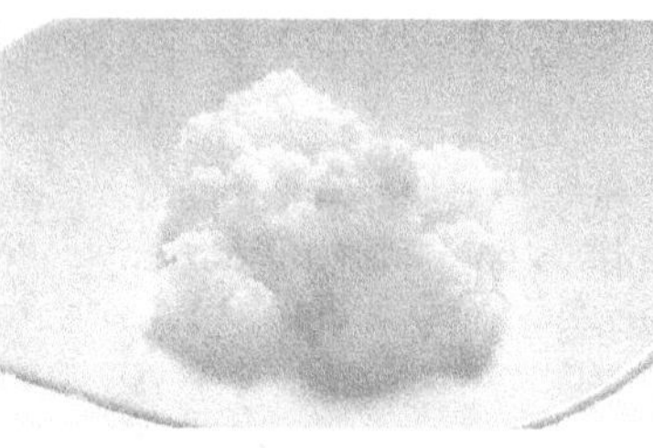

How to make kefir

Making kefir mixed with goat milk is a straightforward
process.

Necessary tools:

- Plastic strainer.
- Plastic spoon.
- Glass jar (traditional milk pint bottle size) with holes
  punctured on the lid for oxygen.

Leave the remainder of the unused goat milk refrigerated.

Pour enough goat milk to fill up 1/3 of the bottle. Place the
kefir grains inside to blend with the milk. Allow the kefir to
fuse with the milk for 24 hours at room temperature. The kefir
granules will prevent the milk from rotting. You will know
what I mean.

24 hours later….

The milk should have become thick, sludge-like and the kefir
granules will float up to the surface. Separate the kefir grains
from the milk by pouring the mixture into a container filtered
by a plastic strainer.

Note: The kefir grains are fragile living organisms. Avoid touching with a metallic object or with fingers.

Place the kefir granules aside. In the plastic strainer, gently rinse the kefir mushrooms with water. Prepare a new kefir mixture to leave for 24 hours. Notice that the kefir granules have multiplied.

Time to drink the kefir-infused milk. Goat milk alone tastes delicious. Kefir mixed with goat milk left for 24 hours at room temperature tastes quite horrible. The taste is sour and smells awful. I like to mix some slices of bananas, and flavored stevia with the kefir drink. If the taste is still intolerable, mix some cocoa together with flavored stevia.

Remember, taste comes last.

Search some videos online on how to make kefir.

Drink kefir mixed with goat milk once or twice a day, permanently. The kefir fused with goat milk will multiply the existing probiotics from the primal defense tablets and continuously add more and regenerate probiotics in the bowels forever.

How do you know if you lack friendly bacteria in the intestines?

If you are unsure of what's going on inside, the best way is to get examined. I have found two powerful methods that can pin down everything that is going on in the system.

How to know what's going on within:

1. Iridology
2. Dark field microscopy (live blood cell analysis)

Iridology is the science of examining the iris, and dark field microscopy is examining a drop of blood under a microscope. Microscopists can be difficult to track and sometimes cannot provide accurate information according to the practitioner's skill level.

I have had better experience with iridologists. Iridology is a strange science, and it pinned down everything that was going wrong with my body. Please check out my intestinal cleanse program for more information.

Summary:

The monstrous physique program is shorter than any of my other books. The reason is because this program is an add-on and cannot function in isolation. In any case, the few extensions outlined in this program will make MONSTROUS differences in your physique!

Let's move onto the workout section…

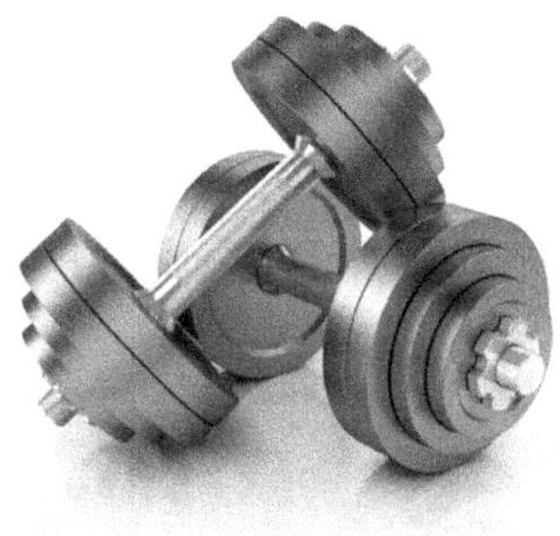

 MONSTROUS WORKOUT

Since you are aiming to build a monstrous physique, I would assume you have some experience lifting weights. The basics of lifting weights are covered in the *How to Build More Muscle than Ever Before* program.

Here I will add a few sage tips to the existing workouts. Obviously, the workouts to build a monstrous physique will be a little more challenging→ but not a lot harder.

Monstrous Workout #1:

Here you will follow the same schedule as the previous bodybuilding program.

Day 1: (chest/triceps/bicep)

Day 2: (legs/glutes)

Day 3: (shoulder/back/lats)

(chest/triceps/bicep)

in order from first to last exercise.

    1   Barbell bench-press (chest)
    2   Dumbbell fly (chest)
    3   Lying close-up barbell triceps (triceps) extension behind the head
    4   Alternate incline dumbbell curl (bicep)

In the monstrous workout, you will add one more exercise to hit the same muscle twice per workout session.

For example:

On chest + triceps + bicep day… pump the triceps or chest x2.

Lying close-up barbell (first) + dumbbell one arm triceps extension (second).

If you do a barbell triceps workout, follow up with a dumbbell exercise, or bodyweight exercise.

Barbell bench-press + Incline barbell bench-press.

This is working out two different muscle groups.

Hit only incline chest or full chest.

Barbell bench-press + pushups.

or

Barbell bench-press + dumbbell press.

By combining pushups with barbell bench press the same muscle will be hit x2.

Adding one more exercise on the same workout day will super-pump one specific muscle group. Believe me, this approach can be tiresome, but you will experience greater results.

Be creative. There are tons of different exercises available. Try out all the exercises, and choose the ones that deliver the best results.

Workout #2 is drop-set. There are many different ways to preform drop-sets, and I have attempted most.

Some personal trainers and gym gurus advise lifting heavy to light, light to heavy; lift all the dumbbells on the rack from lightest to heaviest, do unlimited reps of each, etc.

This approach will overly-exhaust the body and marginally build any measure of muscle mass. I am confident to say that with enough experimentation, I have designed my own drop-set method.

Lifting weights must be rhythmical. Don't lift as much as possible or do as many reps as possible!

Nekoterran's drop-set workout:

Go from heavy to light.

Example bicep drop-set workout:

Begin with…

2 sets of 10 reps

(reach failure with 10 reps)

+

2 sets of 12

(reach failure with 12 reps)

+

1 set of 16

(reach failure with 16 reps)

Finish.

Begin heavy with 2 sets of 10 reps. Then move onto 2 sets of 12 reps. After the heavy sessions are done, do only one set of lighter reps 14-16 reps. You must reach failure with all the reps and sets.

First, you must test out each of the weights to know how many reps you can achieve until failure. Listen to your body.

Drop-sets are more difficult than they sound. Honestly, I like monstrous workout #1. If your body responds better with monstrous workout #2 → stick to #2.

Again, listen to your body. Make your body a friend, not an enemy.

Do not overcomplicate building muscles. To build muscles, the body must burn saturated fats as fuel, be fully colonized with friendly bacteria, have strong digestion, and be fed amino acids to repair/regenerate the muscles after a workout!

Thank you for reading, and enjoy your new monstrous physique!

As an author, I value your reviews. It helps others to make an informed decision before reading the book. If you feel like you have gained enlightened knowledge, please consider leaving a short review in the following link.

It'd be greatly appreciated!

www.nekoterran.com/advice

Thank you and good luck!

Bonus #2: Sign up to receive my future fitness + health products

www.nekoterran.com/advice

All Titles B&W and Color

available at CreateSpace Store…

More Health & Fitness Titles:

Basic Bodybuilding

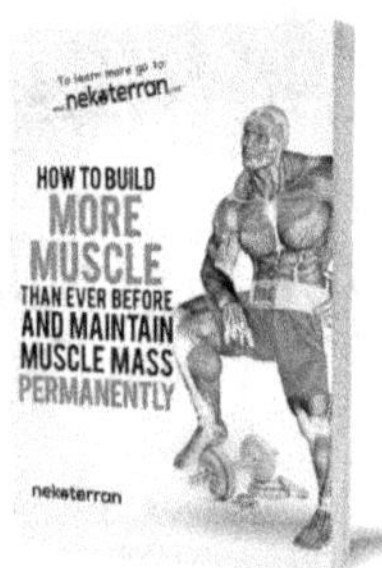

- ✓ What builds muscles.
- ✓ What causes muscle mass deterioration.
- ✓ What causes body fat.
- ✓ How to burn body fat.
- ✓ How to maintain muscle mass.
- ✓ How to maintain a fat-less physique.
- ✓ *Choose only basic bodybuilding or basic weight loss.*

Basic Weight Loss

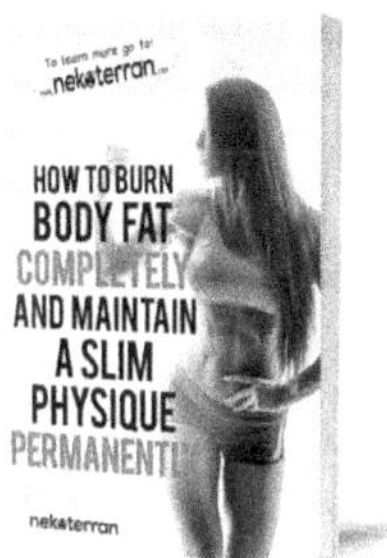

- ✓ What tones/strengthens muscles.
- ✓ What causes muscle mass deterioration.
- ✓ What causes body fat.
- ✓ How to prevent body fat.
- ✓ How to burn existing body fat.
- ✓ How to maintain muscle mass.
- ✓ How to maintain a fat-less physique.
- ✓ *Choose only basic bodybuilding or basic weight loss.*

Basic Internal Detox

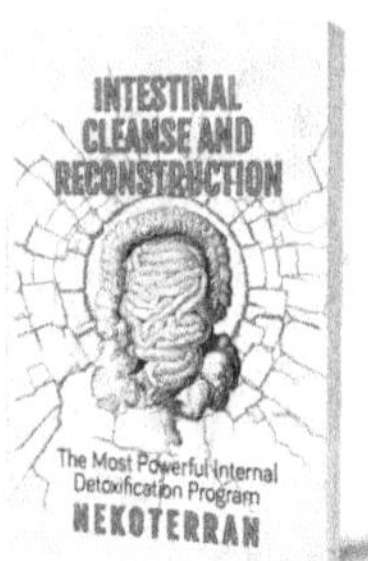

- ✓ Deep internal detoxification program.
- ✓ This is the ideal program to begin with.
- ✓ Complete this program first before attempting weight loss or bodybuilding basics
- ✓ *Works in conjunction with every other program.*

Advanced Bodybuilding

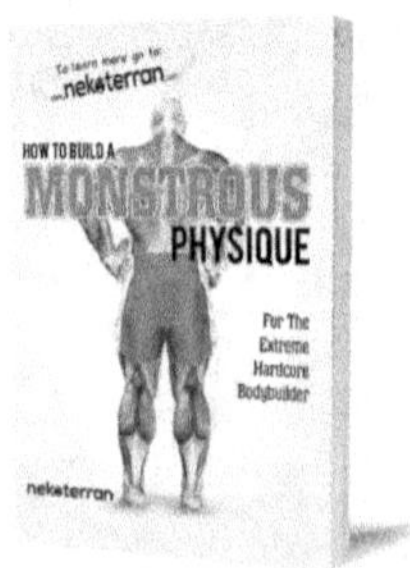

- ✓ For the advanced bodybuilder.
- ✓ The final step out of 3.
- ✓ *Must first complete the internal detox program.*
- ✓ *Must first complete the basic bodybuilding program.*